# Table of Contents

# Disclaimer

This is NOT medical advice. If you are having blood sugar issues/problems, seek medical attention. Consult your physician/medical professional before any diet changes or changes in medicine. I am NOT a doctor or any other health professional including dietician, nutritionist or diabetes educator. This book is for inspirational and entertainment purposes only. I am simply telling you what helped me to lower my blood sugar and A1C as well as healing my kidney damage from type 2 diabetes. Your results may be different.

# Introduction

Hello, I'm Alan King.  I was diagnosed as a type 2 diabetic with kidney damage in November 2021. My glucose reading was 329 and my hba1c was 12.9 (nondiabetics have an A1C below 5.7).  I thought, "There goes 95% of my diet, what do I eat now?" A diabetes educator gave me some info but after reading the recommended diet, (from the ADA. They recommended ¼ of my plate be carbs and pictured was a baked potato) decided against following that diet.  It was filled with too many carbs and starches (I had learned in junior high school that carbs turn to sugar as soon as they hit your stomach).  Carbs & starches are a diabetic's enemy (like a poison).  So I started an internet search.  There I found the Beat Diabetes channel, Dr. Jason Fung and Dr. Richard Bernstein.  They offered fantastic advice on how to beat diabetes. There were other channels that offered the same bad advice as the diabetes educator (i.e. sweet potatoes are better than white potatoes, brown rice not white rice etc.). But the Beat Diabetes channel, Dr. Fung and Dr. Bernstein (via their You Tube channels) helped me to get my blood sugar levels down to normal within a few months.  Their advice was low carbs, intermittent fasting/time restricted eating, read labels on food packages and TEST, TEST,

TEST with my blood sugar meter. I check my blood sugar one hour and then again two hours after my meals. The reason is to find out which food item is causing any blood sugar spikes to go over 139 mg/dl. Today my hba1c is 5.3 and my blood sugar readings fall within non diabetic range. Even after meals.

The reason I am so passionate about beating type 2 diabetes is that it runs on both sides of my family. I have seen some of those family members suffer and some have passed away prematurely with a lot of serious medical issues due to diabetes complications. Not to mention friends and co-workers.

I look at it this way, if someone has a nut allergy the medical advice is to stop eating nuts, if someone is gluten or lactose intolerant, stop your intake of gluten or lactose. It just makes sense to me since a diabetic is carbohydrate intolerant, stop the carbs. It's that simple.

I have found that there are a lot of naysayers & fear mongers, including some in the medical community. I decided that it is my body and quality of life. It is ME that will suffer not the naysayers and fear mongers.

The diet that I am on is my permanent way of eating & way of life. I know that I cannot go back to the standard American diet. I'll just continue to eat fat, a **moderate** amount of protein, fiber and drastically reduced carb meals.  YES, these meals can be maintained.  I have included some recipes in this book along with a few meal ideas.  There are plenty of low carb/keto recipe channels on You Tube that I have found.  So go to You Tube and search for low carb and keto recipes of your favorite meals.

I have found that I beat my type 2 diabetes in five easy steps.  1. Drastically cut carbs, starches & sugar from my diet, including natural sugars.  2. Eliminated ALL grains (no one needs oat meal including steel cut oats, corn or bread, white, brown or whole wheat etc.).  3. Removed all vegetable/seed oils. 4. Ate more fatty meat, like red meat, poultry and fish. 5. Exercised more.  I explain more about these steps in this book and what I have learned on my journey.

I have included some of the websites, You Tube channels and books where I found my information to beat diabetes.  Results may vary.

# Section 1

# What I Did to Beat Diabetes

And

**Things I Wished I Knew When 1ˢᵗ Diagnosed**

# Safe Foods

READ ingredients (the fine print for hidden sugars, carbs and starches) on food and drink packages as well as the nutritional information. These foods and food products won't spike blood sugar or very little. Always check your blood sugar before, 1 hour and then again 2 hours after every meal. By doing this you will find what foods are safe for you to eat. I let my meter decide what my diet is. Remember to TEST! See what your meter says. Don't take anyone's word for it. Check your blood sugar to see for yourself. This is just a partial list:

- Asparagus
- Cream Cheese
- Broccoli
- Parmesan Cheese
- Cabbage
- Cauliflower
- Sardines
- Cucumbers
- Tuna

- Eggplan
- Cod Fish
- Bell Pepper
- Trout
- Mushrooms
- Beef
- Zucchini
- Chicken (un-breaded)
- Anything low carb/high fiber

- Arugula
- Spinach
- Mayonnaise (made from avocado)
- Pork
- Sour Cream
- Turkey
- Mustard
- Lamb
- Vinegar
- Bison
- Soy Sauce
- Deer/Venison
- Butter, grass feed
- Almond Milk (unsweet)
- Extra Virgin Olive Oil
- Unsweet Chocolate
- MCT Oil
- Almond Flour, unsweet
- Coconut Flour, unsweet
- Block Cheese, no pre-shredded
- Decaf Coffee
- Lemon Water (from freshly squeezed lemons)

# FYI

Broccoli, bitter melon and okra have been known to assist in lowering glucose in the blood. Not only have I read about it I have personally experienced it. For me broccoli works better raw, maybe lightly steamed. Be sure to include these vegetables in your salads and low carb meals. On occasion I will sprinkle flax seed on my salads and other meals.

There are other foods that assist in lowering glucose. Test them individually if you would like.

According to www.healthline.com/leading-casues-of-death, diabetes is the 7th leading cause of death (Their info was taken from the CDC's 2021 report). Other leading causes of death include heart disease & stroke. When a person is diabetic, their risk greatly increases for strokes & heart disease. I'm curious to know how many of those that died from strokes & heart disease had diabetes.

# Don't Eat

I don't eat these foods. Just some of the foods are listed. Think low carb (similar to keto). I included both simple and complex carbohydrates on this list. TEST to see what works for you. Maybe some in extreme moderation will be ok. Again, ALWAYS TEST! Let your blood sugar meter decide what you can or cannot eat.

- Sugar
- Margarine
- Potatoes
- Canola Oil
- Sweet Potatoes
- Sunflowers Oil
- Rice (including Brown Rice)
- Peanut Oil
- Soy Milk
- Vegetable Oil
- Bread, all flour or grain base
- Pre-Shredded Cheese (has maltodextrin)
- Artificial sweeteners

- (has maltodextrin)
- Honey
- Low Carb Ice Cream (a keto brand is ok for me)
- Soy Products
- Milk
- Most Fruits
- Most Citrus
- Corn (is a grain not a vegetable)

This is just a partial list. Again, ALWAYS read the ingredients list on the package/label. Anything that spikes my blood sugar meter reading more than 139 mg/dl I have eliminated from my diet.

Feel free to use your glucose meter to test any of these foods individually if you would like. You could get a different result. If you do test, take a pretest just before then a test 30 minutes after your last bite. Do this every 30 minutes for 2 ½ hours. Record your test results. As stated above, I eliminate any foods that spike my blood sugar more than 139 mg/dL.

# Spices/Seasonings/Herbs

Be very careful of seasonings. Some seasonings are ok. Even the same seasoning packaged by a different company can have added ingredients that spike blood sugar. I have found that powdered onion and garlic powder/salt runs my blood sugar up. It didn't matter which brand I used. There might or might not be nutrition/ingredients labels on seasoning packages.  They are not required to by the United States govt.  Go to USDA.gov for more info. So test, test and test!

# Diabetes Is Not Progressive

As long as a person eats a low carb/low spike diet, exercise and with time restricted eating/intermittent fasting, diabetes will reverse for most T2 & pre diabetics.  It did for me and many others.  My kidney damage has also reversed and is normal now.  This was confirmed by blood test from the doctor's office.

# One Meal a Day/OMAD

Occasionally having one meal a day does help me keep my blood sugar low.  I do OMAD several times a month.  I'll have a carnivore meal or maybe a salad or other almost zero carb meal on those days.  It gives my pancreas & beta cells time to rest. There will be more about this later.

# Time Restricted
# Eating/Intermittent Fasting

Time restricted eating helped me also.  I have two meals a day spaced 4 to 6 hours apart. I have my last meal of the day no later than 6:30-7 p.m. If I eat past that time it raises my morning glucose reading, even though it was a low carb meal. I have bulletproof coffee for breakfast.  Usually two cups, sometimes three.  This is enough to keep me satiated until lunch time around 1 or 2 p.m.  Most of the time, I do 16/8.  That's an eight hour window of eating and 16 hours fasting.  Remember this, 8 of those 16 hours of fasting is done while sleeping.  Then I will have bulletproof coffee for breakfast.  One of the reasons one needs I.F. or Time Restricted Eating is to give your body time to rest & heal.

# Bulletproof Coffee

In your favorite coffee cup, put one or two table spoon(s) of heavy whipping cream and water if instant, grass fed butter, coconut oil or MCT oil and decaf coffee.  Heat and enjoy.

# Be Careful of Books Magazines & the Internet

Be very careful on the internet and with books & magazines.  There is a lot of false/misleading information out there. If they say count calories to lower glucose & not carbs tells me they know very little, probably nothing about lowering glucose. Make sure that any information found you TEST! I also discovered that some of the keto recipes don't always work and after testing, have to make adjustments to them. I have listed some of the ones that work for me later in this book.

# Exercise

Walking shortly after my meals really helps lower my blood sugar.  The more brisk the walk the better my results will be. Any exercise that gets my heart rate up, including lifting weights/building muscle mass forces sugar into my cells without the help or need of insulin.  Exercise is no reason to purposely eat high carb/starchy food items.  Then say, "I'll walk it off." It doesn't work that way.

# Resistant Starch

Resistant starch is the cooling/freezing high carb foods for a period of time (usually overnight). They say the carbs become "safe" then. I have only had moderate luck with resistant starch. What I have found for the most part, rice is still rice, pasta is still pasta & potatoes are still potatoes.  Test for yourself.  You might get a different result.  They're no two diabetics exactly the same.

# Net Carbs

Net carbs usually do work for me.  Net carbs is subtracting the grams of fiber & sugar alcohols from the total carbs and the result is the net carbs. But be careful of prepackaged products such as keto breads and other packaged keto products.  If you're a newly diagnosed diabetic, I wouldn't do net carbs until your blood sugar is under control and hba1c is below 5.7.  Just go by total carbs until then.

# Alcoholic Drinks

Stay away from alcoholic drinks.  Alcoholic drinks could interfere with diabetic medications & make insulin resistance worse among other things.  As always, consult your medical professional.

# Caffeine

It has been shown that caffeine can raise blood sugar and insulin levels in your blood.  Caffeine can lower insulin sensitivity in cells also. Therefore, over time, could make your diabetes worse. This happens to some diabetics faster than others.  Decaf is better although it is not 100% caffeine free.

# Log Meals/Meter Readings

I keep a log of my blood sugar readings and what my meals consist of.  That way I can tell what is safe and what the food does to my blood sugar. Over time you will be able to tell what you can safely eat or not eat.  Your doctor will appreciate you keeping a log of your blood sugar readings & your meals.

# Naked Carbs/Food Order

I have had very little luck in dressing high carb foods with fats along with the order I eat my foods.

That means not having an avocado with a glazed donut or bacon/sausage on any kind of bread (white, brown or sourdough). It will not matter which you eat first.  Expect your blood sugar to go into orbit. This goes for ANY mixing of extremely high carb foods with fats. Dressing **moderate** carb food items with fiber & fat usually works for me.  The best is to stay low carb with as much fiber as you can get with all food items. Your results may vary.  TEST and see what works for you.

# GI Index/Glycemic Load

Neither the glycemic index chart OR the glycemic load chart alone worked for me.  Be very careful of the foods on these two charts.  As always TEST, TEST, TEST!  Take NO ONE'S word for it!  No matter what or who they are or the initials beside their name.  See what works for you.  Again, one size does NOT fit all!   Like some medical, dieticians & nutritionist seem to imply with those charts

# Dawn Effect/
# Dawn Phenomenon

This is your blood sugar reading you get when you first wake up of a morning.  The reading is usually higher at that time of day because of hormones waking you up.  The dawn effect can last way up into the morning, sometimes until around noon. How I keep my dawn effect within the normal morning range is I don't eat anything past 7 p.m. the previous evening.  The earlier you eat your evening meal the better, between 5pm & 6 pm.  I don't drink diet sodas past that time either (rarely will I drink them anyway).  Water is best but on occasion an unsweetened decaf tea or black decaf coffee is ok late in the evening.  It took me several weeks to get my morning blood sugar readings to normal.  Don't give up.  Give it time.  I keep my morning fasting glucose reading below 100 mg/dl.

# Somogyi Effect

The Somogyi effect is not the same as the Dawn Phenomenon.  For example, a person can take their insulin at bedtime and still wake up with high blood sugar.  This is believed to happen with T1D > T2D.  This effect could be problems with your diabetes management.  Consult your physician if this is happening to you and for more information.  So far I have not experienced this effect.

# False Lows

A false low is when you feel the symptoms of low blood sugar but it is actually not low but normal.  The body has gotten used to high blood sugar and when it goes back to normal, it can seem as if you might be having a hypo.  It is like getting in a hot shower and then when you get out you feel cold.  Your body will adjust.  Remember, you did not have hypo symptoms when your blood sugar readings were normal. Your body just "forgot" what normal blood sugar feels like. That feeling is only temporary. If you have any questions, consult your physician.

# Blood Sugar Levels Chart

|  | Normal | Pre-Diabetic | Type 2 |
|---|---|---|---|
| Fasting | 70-99 mg/dl | 100-124 mg/dl | 126 mg/dl or more |
| 2 Hours After Meals | <140mg/dl | 140-199 mg/dl | 200 mg/dl or more |

# Sample Daily Menu

| Breakfast | 2 cups of bullet proof coffee |
|---|---|
| Lunch (Between 1 & 2 p.m.) | Salad with Ranch Dressing (full fat) or 2 to 3 ground beef patties and green beans |
| Supper/Dinner | Meat (no bread coating) & 1-2 low carb vegetables |

Maybe an occasional low carb dessert right after supper/dinner on the weekends will be ok.

This is the menu I use.  The earlier your dinner or supper the better it is.  No snacking for the rest of the day.  No diet sodas either.  As stated earlier, water, unsweetened tea or black coffee is ok to drink.

More recipes are in Section 2.

# Apple Cider Vinegar

What some diabetics do is mix 1 table spoon of raw, unfiltered, organic acv with mother into an 8 ounce glass of water before their meals.  According to some research, by doing this it helps blunt any sugar spikes and slow down digestion.  The studies also suggest that it could help with weight loss too.  I tried it once or twice but found that it was too acidic for me.  I know some T2's that have had positive results with it.  If you try it, TEST, TEST, TEST. Do this before your meals and after.

# 6 Small Meals a Day

I don't see any point in doing this.  Every time a person eats, it raises blood sugar & insulin. Frequent meals could keep one's A1C elevated.  It will be very difficult for your glucose to go back to baseline, if it even does.  Frequent meals also will require more & more insulin (hyperinsulinemia, go to www.my.clevelandclinic.org/health/diseases/2417

for more info) and could possibly make insulin resistance worse including in T1's.  Too much insulin also causes weight gain & can be problematic in other ways too.  The best is to have 2 meals in a 6 to 8 hour window.  No snacks either.  If you have a highly physical job or you're very active, you might need more carbs to keep from having a hypoglycemia incident.  Talk with your doctor about all of these things.

# Stress/Sleep

When a person is stressed, it raises the "stress" hormone cortisol.  Avoid stressful situations as much as possible.  Getting enough sleep is essential, a must.  Do all you can to get enough sleep.

# Studies/Research

Be careful of studies/research about diabetes and what foods to eat or not eat.  I have found that some of those studies are paid for by food and pharmaceutical companies (look at an organization's major donors list).  Some of the results, therefore, appear to lean in their favor.  They're biased in other words.  That is one more reason to test. ALWAYS TEST! Again, don't take anyone's word for it.  No matter whom they are or claim to be, especially on the internet and authors of books. Pay attention to the way the tests were conducted. Were the tests observational, did they have a control group or was the test conducted using a questionnaire? Seems to me the research/studies with a control group would be more scientific. Definitely no questionnaire studies should be considered.

# Because "They" Want My Numbers Higher Than Normal

Remember it is YOU that will suffer the consequences of higher than normal blood sugar. Not the doctor, dietitian, nutritionist or diabetes educator. NOT A SINGLE ONE OF THEM. It is your eyes & kidneys. You're the one that could have amputation(s) of toes & other limbs. This includes development of neuropathy, strokes & heart attacks. I started going to another doctor shortly after being diagnosed for this reason (he was satisfied with higher than normal numbers A1C > 5.6). Currently, I am under the care of a doctor (I see every 3 months for blood test and a diabetic checkup) that believes in low carb/low starches and exercise to crush diabetes. And that is exactly what has happened to me. Again, my kidney injury has also gone away. No signs of it at all. EVERY diabetic, from 5 to 105, has a right to have normal blood sugar levels (A1C<5.7). Health professionals don't always agree on treatment. Some are still "old school" treating the symptoms but not the cause (for most T2's & pre diabetics is having insulin resistance).  So be careful and choose your doctor wisely.

# Online hbA1c Calculators

I use two online A1C calculators.  As stated above, my doctor orders blood work every three months including an A1C test.  The reason I use online A1C calculators is so I can make adjustments to my diet if I need to before my doctor's appointment.  I take the average of about 40 days of "Mike the meter" glucose test from my log.  The online calculators that I use are listed below:

www.jennybrown.net/Calculators/A1ccalc3.php

https://professional.diabetes.org/diapro/glucose_cal. This one is from the ADA.

# Health Professionals Do Not Always Agree On Diets

Since I was diagnosed, I have also found that health professionals do not always agree on a diabetic's diet either.  There's some that say to do the ADA diet plan (ok to eat higher carbs), some low carb others vegan/vegetarian or natural foods.  Still, others say everything in moderation or replace refined carbs with complex carbs and you'll be fine. Also some say no keto recipes others say yes. I have found that for me it's the low carb, low spike diet with some "clean" keto recipes.

# Hypoglycemia/Low Blood Sugar

Hypoglycemia or a Hypo is when a person's blood sugar falls below 70mg/dl (3.9 mmol/L).  Here are some of the symptoms:

| | | |
|---|---|---|
| Headache | Fast Heart Rate | Seizure |
| Feeling Tired | Sweating | Shakiness |
| Clumsy | Feeling Nervous | Death |
| Trouble talking | Hunger | |
| Confusion | Passing Out | |

If you feel any of these symptoms (can be only one), check your glucose a.s.a.p.  I always carry my glucose meter with me everywhere I go.  Also, always have a soda, candy or something that will run your blood sugar up fast with you at all times. I was advised, when I was first diagnosed, to keep a regular non diet soda in the refrigerator at all times. Just in case.

# Hyperglycemia/High Blood Sugar

Here are some of the symptoms of high blood sugar. A person does not have to have all of these symptoms.  These are the most common:

| | |
|---|---|
| Fatigue / Weakness | Numbness in hands / Feet |
| Blurry Vision | Increased Urination |
| Always Thirsty | |
| Wounds that are slow / Wont Heal | Nausea / Vomiting |
| | Fruity Breath |
| Weight Loss / Gain | Always Hungry |

These symptoms are for type 1 and type 2. Other types of diabetes include MODY, LADA (type 1.5) & GESTATIONAL (women only) that could have some of these symptoms. Get checked if you have any of these symptoms.  As stated above, one does not have to have all of these symptoms, a lot of people only notice one or two.  Or someone might think their symptom(s) are related to working an off shift at their job.  I thought the symptoms I had was due to working nights.  My diabetes was found while being checked for something else. Usually an A1C test is given to help determine if you are diabetic.  See your doctor.

## Signs of Insulin Resistance

- Dark Rough Skin under armpits, back & sides of neck (acanthosis nigricans or just nigricans)
- Skin Tags (small skin growths that might resemble warts)

- Eye/Sight Changes
- Any of the Symptoms of High Blood Sugar (See Hyperglycemia list above)

If you have any of these conditions or symptoms, go to your doctor and get checked asap.  It could be insulin resistance starting up or you already have it. Not everyone that has or is developing insulin resistance will have skin tags or acanthosis nigricans but may have symptom(s) of high blood sugar.

# Low Glucose Trumps Nutritional Food Items

It doesn't matter if the food item is extremely nutritional if it runs your glucose up to the moon and back. As stated earlier, the extra sugar in a diabetic's blood (glycation) is what causes the damage to internal organs, blood veins & vessels as well as nerve damage. Nerve damage can cause amputations, neuropathy, strokes, heart attacks, & E.D. in men.  Premature death can also occur. Refer to the SAFE FOODS section of this book and you should get plenty of nutrition while keeping your glucose low.

# When to Check Blood Sugar

A lot of health professionals say to check your blood sugar once or twice a day or maybe two hours after every meal only (but what if you peak 1 hour after?). My question is, how will you know what is safe to eat without having sky high blood sugar? One needs to find their peak. To find out what is safe to eat and when you peak, check your blood sugar just before your meal, 30 minutes after your last bite. Then again, one hour after you finish your meal. Do this every 30 minutes for 2 ½ to 3 hours. By doing it this way you find out when and how high your blood sugar peaks and starts to return to your pre meal test. I eliminate any food that causes my meter reading to be 139 mg/dl (damage starts > than 140 mg/dl). After you have been doing it this way for a while, you will learn what you can eat and not eat. Then it won't be necessary to test so much. I only test that much if I am trying a new low carb/keto recipe. Otherwise I test one hour then again 2 hours after I finish my meal. I don't trust the GI Index or the Glycemic Load list. That's like saying "one size fits all". Well, it DOES NOT fit all. Everyone is a little different in their degree of insulin resistance. I also test upon waking up of a morning and just before going to bed. I don't want to go to sleep if I am unknowingly near a hypo. So TEST at those times too.

# Buddy System

Find someone that's diabetic also and both of you can be responsible to each other.  It's much easier when you have a partner.  It's even better if you're the same type diabetic.  There's more about this later.

# Recommended Books

Diabetes Code by Dr. Jason Fung, Diabetes Code Cookbook by Dr. Jason Fung, Dr. Bernstein's Diabetes Solution by Dr. Richard Bernstein, You Can Achieve Normal Blood Sugar, 60 Ways to Lower Your Blood Sugar both by Dennis Pollock, Blood Sugar 101 by Jenny Ruhl, Lies My Doctor Told Me by Ken D. Berry, MD, FAAFP and books by Dr. Robert Atkins.

# Click Like & Subscribe Channels

Beat Diabetes, Sugar High, Dr. Eric Westman, Ken D Berry MD, Jason Fung, Health Coach Kait, Dr. Sarah Hallberg, Dr. Eric Berg, Dr. Sten Ekberg, Diet Doctor, Dr. Benjamin (Ben) Bikman, The Habits Doctor, Jay Sampat, Type One Talks, Type Rhino, Dr. Willie Ong & Dee Dang (both Tagalog).

# Insulin Resistance

Being insulin resistant is the key player in being a type 2 and pre-diabetic. Insulin's job is to "push" the sugar into your cells from your blood after your meals.  Ones cells become resistant to the insulin, there's too much of it. Your cells then say, "We have had enough" and will stop accepting the sugar from the insulin. Cells become immune to it in other words.  Insulin also sends signals to your liver to store the extra sugar so your body can use it later.  It will take longer and longer for your blood sugar to go back down to baseline. Also, insulin resistance has been linked to women with PCOS. For more detailed information go to these websites, www.webmd.com, www.cdc.gov, www.mayoclinic.org, www.diabetes.org or ask your physician.

# Metabolic Syndrome

Metabolic syndrome (now known as insulin resistance) is when several conditions happen inside your body at the same time (including a fatty liver & pancreas). The conditions that happen can increase the risk of heart attacks, heart disease, pre diabetes, type 2 diabetes and strokes just to mention a few.  For more information you can visit this website, www.mayoclinic.org and talk with your physician.

# Weight Loss Diets & Diabetic Diets

Weight loss diets are designed just for that.  To shed pounds.  Some of the weight loss diets might have sugars and carbohydrates (although some not as much) in them as a lot of them count calories instead.  Those diets still have too many carbs, sugars and starches for a diabetic.  The ketogenic or keto diet is a weight loss diet.  But a diabetic can eat "clean" keto meals & recipes. Don't do the official keto diet unless your physician/health care professional prescribes it to you.

# Diet/No Sugar Added/Sugar Free/Zero Sugar Products

Beware of prepackaged products marked as such. A lot of these products could still have added sugars of some type or starches, flour, carbohydrates or sweeteners that do. Look for anything that can raise blood sugar or turn to sugar after you eat them. This includes diet drinks of all kinds that have any of these phrases written on the label or package. Be careful of keto products too.  Read ingredients, not just the nutritional information, on EVERY packaged food & drink product.

# Test Strips, Glucose Meters & CGM's

One can get meters and test strips for around $20 or less.  They don't have to be the more expensive brands. Also your physician can write a prescription for these items and your insurance company will cover a large part of the cost, if not free to you. CGM's are prescription required. Check with your doctor. Just be sure to wash & dry your hands thoroughly before you test. By not doing so could interfere with the result.

# Eating Out at Restaurants

Will a diabetic have to give up eating out? Simple answer is no. There's more to it of course. Read the menu checking for low carb/non starchy foods and meals (look for ways to make the meal low carb). One of the restaurants that I found safe for me is Mexican. One can order a steak or chicken fajita meal. Just don't eat the rice and beans or the wrap that might come with it. Another from a Mexican restaurant is a taco salad. Don't eat the shell it comes in and I have already said no beans or rice. Guacamole should be ok. Of course any meat (no sauces, seasonings or bread coating) is ok. Ordering at other types of restaurants is similar. Read the menu & look for low carb foods or ways to make it low carb. Un-breaded meat and a low carb/low starch vegetable or two should be fine. Just be careful of any sauces or seasonings that might be on the vegetables also. I have eaten at a Chinese restaurant and the golden arches with success. Sometimes I will order a breakfast of eggs, tomatoes and two pieces of turkey sausage (no more than two). Just remember low carb, portion size and TEST.

# Natural Foods/Natural Sugar/Natural Ingredients

Overall whole foods are preferred over packaged/processed food products. But not all whole/natural foods are created equal for someone with blood sugar issues. For example, spinach is a natural food. It is loaded with all kinds of vitamins and minerals, low in carbs/starches and won't spike blood sugar. Another natural food, potatoes including sweet potatoes, has vitamins and minerals a person needs but the carbs & starches in them will spike blood sugar to the stratosphere. Just because a food product is labelled natural it does not mean that a diabetic can safely eat it. This includes most fruits & citrus (a lot have fructose, a sugar) of many different kinds. Take the time to learn about a food's ingredients.

## Full Fat, Fat Free, Reduced Fat

If the fat is reduced or taken out of a processed food product, they have to compensate for the loss of flavor/taste with something. It is usually some kind of sugar they use, high in carbs. Take a bottle of ranch salad dressing for example. Full fat salad dressing will have less carbs, in ranch dressing one or two carbs per serving. Fat free or reduced fat will have several carbs (because of the sugar). This is done on most of the "fat free" food products I have compared. Read the labels and compare for yourself. Avoid the bad fats such as hydrogenated fats, margarine, artificial trans-fats, deep fried foods etc.  Other fats are good.  They help make you feel full after a meal.  Always read ingredients.

## One Does Not Have to Starve to Lower A1C/Blood Sugar

One does not have to go hungry to lower their blood sugar/A1C.  The answer is simple.  Just eat more when you do eat.  For example, if you have a beef patty and green beans and you're still hungry have another beef patty or two until you are satiated. Do remember portion control.  This is what I do (I usually have 4 beef patties).  Doing it this way works with about any low carb food.  Remember that you are on a diabetic diet not a weight loss diet.  Also keep in mind that too much protein can raise glucose also.

## Why Sugar Stays High Without Eating Sugar/Carbs

One's liver (and kidneys to a lesser degree) can make too much sugar/glucose from non carb sources. Those sources include proteins, ketones and fats. This process is regulated by insulin.  For people that do not have any insulin (T1's) or are insulin resistant (pre diabetics & T2's) your liver will think (because of fluctuations in hormones) your body needs more and more glucose. This is known as gluconeogenesis.  This condition may not get better in just two or three days of fasting. One needs to continue to fast, exercise and lose weight. One still can be "skinny" and still have fat around their internal organs (liver, pancreas & stomach) known as belly fat or visceral fat. It's a part of metabolic syndrome.

I will experience, to some degree, gluconeogenesis from time to time (even though I don't have too much visceral fat) because of the fluctuations in hormones. I will go all day with higher blood sugar even though my meals are extremely low carb with little to no variations in my routine. What I have found is to continue my routine and maybe will do OMAD (one meal a day) for a day or two. The meal that I will have on my OMAD days is carnivore, consisting of three or four beef patties or baked/rotisserie chicken, maybe an omelet or a salad. Along with brisk exercise, this makes my cells absorb the excess glucose my liver is producing.

I will add that gluconeogenesis is a natural process. It helps prevent hypoglycemia between meals. The brain and certain other organs need glucose. In my experience it's my insulin resistance and occasional low blood sugar ($< 70$ mg/dL) when my liver produces a greater amount of sugar because it "thinks" (because of hormones sending signals) I don't have enough glucose for my cells, because of insulin resistance, my cells won't accept the excess glucose.

For more information, go to this website: www.ncbi.nlm.nih.gov/books/NBK544346/ or speak with your doctor.

## Soleus Push Up

This exercise is performed sitting down. It works out the soleus muscle in the calf. The soleus push up will force glucose into your cells without the need of insulin rather quickly. If you are at a desk all day or have a sedentary life style, you can do this exercise and no one will know you're exercising. It can be done at the dinner table at Grandma's house this Thanksgiving or Christmas. To perform this exercise, sit down with your legs at approximately a 90 degree angle. Lift your heels up as high as you can while keeping your toes and the ball of your feet on the floor. After you lift your heels, hold tightly for a second or so then repeat. Do this for about 10 to 15 minutes. I do about three sets of 50 and it works. This exercise will work for T1's too.

# Different Diets for Diabetic Types

Type 1's might have a different diet plan than type 2's. While T2's and pre diabetics are insulin resistant, a T1, in theory, is not. A T1 does not produce insulin (they inject it) and T2's do. Therefore, a T1 can, again in theory, eat higher carb foods than a type 2. A T1 can benefit from a low carb diet (less insulin needed) but a T2 may not benefit from a T1 diet.  Be aware of the differences in all of the types of diabetes.  Keep this in mind if you're doing the buddy system previously mentioned on page 12.

## Diabetic Drugs One Should NEVER Take Sulfonylureas (SU)
Glimepiride, Glyburide and Glipizide

What are sulfonylureas?  The sulfonylureas class of medications includes (most common & their generic names) glimepiride, glyburide and glipizide. They are a class of diabetic medications for type 2's only because a type 1 does not produce insulin. There are other medications in this class.

How do they work?  They work by "forcing" the beta cells in a type 2's pancreas to produce more and more insulin, eventually causing the beta cells to self-destruct or beta cell apoptosis.  How fast this happens depends on the person. Because a type 2 diabetic could already have some beta cell burn out, this could happen pretty quickly. When it does happen, the body will for all practical purposes will become an insulin dependent type one diabetic. Another reason is this class of medications can cause hypoglycemia and weight gain. There are several other unwanted side effects.  Talk with your doctor for more information.

**Section 2**


# Low Carb/Keto

# Recipes

# &

# Meal Ideas

## Breakfast Food Recipes & Ideas
Good anytime of the day.

### Chaffles/Low Carb Waffles

1 cup of shredded mozzarella cheese
2 eggs

Instructions:

Pre heat waffle maker.
Shred 1 cup (125 grams) of mozzarella cheese.
In a medium size bowl, crack two eggs and mix
with the shredded cheese until mixed.
Place half of the mixture on the waffle iron.  When
the waffle iron quits steaming, it is done.
Place the other half of the mixture on the waffle
iron and repeat.
This recipe makes two large waffles.
(Optional)  You can put any low carb topping on it
you wish.  I put grass fed butter and sometimes sour
cream on mine.

I do not have the macros.  I have tested this recipe
and for me, only a minimal spike.  Again, always
TEST yourself.


# Maple Syrup/Low Carb/Keto/No Sugar

2 cups of water
1.5 cups brown Swerve brand sweetener
½ tsp xanthan gum
¼ tsp salt
(optional) ½ tsp vanilla extract
1 tsp maple extract

In a medium saucepan, on medium low heat, put the

2 cups of water, bring water to a simmer.  Then mix together the Swerve, xanthan gum and salt.  When the water starts to simmer, start adding the mixture a little at a time.  Do not mix vigorously or the sweetener will crystallize.  After you mix the ingredients, simmer on low for 3 to 4 minutes.  When you take it off the stove, this is when the maple extract and vanilla extract (optional) is added.  Transfer to the container of your choice.  I keep an old syrup bottle for mine.  It can be kept in the refrigerator for about a week.  The brown Swerve will crystalize but you can use a strainer on the next use.

## Scrambled/Fried/Omelets/Hard Boiled Eggs

Scramble or Fry 2 eggs. Use real grass fed butter to scramble or fry the eggs in.  For boiled eggs, boil on high for at least 15-16 minutes in plenty of water.

2-3 slices of tomatoes.  If the tomatoes are large, just use 2 slices.

 Use only ½ of a large avocado.  If the avocado is small a whole one is ok.

Sprinkle all items with flax seed or flax meal.

For an **omelet**, you can put in broccoli and sliced mushrooms or any very low carb vegetables.  Some people put in slices of bitter melon or eggplant also.  It has been shown that bitter melon can help lower blood sugar. It does for me.

# Cereal, Low Carb/Keto

In a small bowl, mix unsweetened coconut flakes, pecan pieces, walnut pieces and slivered almonds. It's ok to leave out what you don't like.

Put unsweetened almond milk over it

Enjoy.

You can substitute the unsweetened almond milk with 1 part heavy whipping cream and three parts water.

# Toast/Bread

Ingredients for Low Carb Bread/Toast:

1.5 cups almond flour, 2 Tablespoons coconut flour, 2 Tablespoons baking powder, 6 eggs and ¾ cup extra virgin olive oil.  (Optional) 1 Tablespoon sour cream

Directions:
Preheat oven to 375 degrees F.  1. Line your loaf

pan with parchment paper.  2. Whisk all ingredients in a medium bowl until combined.  3. Pour batter into a 9x5 loaf pan ¾ full. Then shake or tap loaf pan to get any air bubbles out.  4. Bake for about 30 minutes or until tooth pick comes out clean.  Allow to cool before slicing.  6. Slice and then toast however you toast regular bread.

# Biscuits & Gravy Low Carb

## Ingredients

2 1/4 cups almond flour
1 tsp cream of tartar
1 tsp of baking powder
6 egg whites
4 tbls cold unsalted butter

## Directions

Add almond flour to a food processor
Add the egg whites
Add salt, cream of tartar then baking powder
Close lid and give a few pulses to combine.  Then add butter.  Give and few more pulses to combine in the butter into the mixture.
Line baking sheet with parchment paper.  Divide into seven to nine biscuits (depending on size). Bake at 400*f for 12 to 24 minutes or until golden brown.  Keep checking on them after 12 minutes.

Almond flour can burn easy.    All ovens vary. Recipe can be cut in half for less.

## Gravy

1 Tbls butter
2 cups heavy whipping cream
1 cup water
¼ tsp xanthan gum
¼ tsp salt
1 tsp salt


## Directions

With the stove eye on high, melt the butter
Add ingredients in order
Reduce heat to medium
Stir mixture for 10-15 minutes until it is as thick as you want it


I have tested this recipe and it works with minimal spike.  These two recipes can be found on Papa G's You Tube channel.  For more low carb/keto recipes, click like and subscribe to Papa G's You Tube channel.

## Low Carb Pancakes

### Ingredients

3 eggs, small to medium
3 tbls heavy whipping cream
3 tbls olive oil
3 tbls unsweetened coconut flour
½ tsp salt
½ tsp of baking powder
½ tsp swerve

## Directions

In a medium bowl, mix all the ingredients together until a batter is formed.  At a slightly lower temperature, cook the pancakes like they're regular based pancakes.

Just double the recipe for more.

# Doughnuts

## Ingredients

2 Tbls coconut flour
6 Tbls almond flour
1 Tbls xanthan gum
½ tsp of baking powder
2 Tbls of low carb sweetener of choice.  I use Swerve.

In a second bowl put your wet ingredients.

2 Tbls of coconut oil, melted
2 large eggs

Directions

Pre Heat oven to 350 degrees.  Stir dry ingredients
in the same bowl.  Then in a second bowl, melt the
coconut oil then put the eggs in and stir.  Then mix
the wet and dry ingredients, stir until combined.
Put in your pre heated oven for around 20 minutes.
Due to variance in ovens check on them after 10 to
15 minutes.

Makes about 4 cake like doughnuts.  For more just
double the recipe. Glaze recipe is on the next page.

# Glaze for the Donuts

## Ingredients

¼ cup of unsalted butter
¼ cup of heavy whipping cream
½ cup of powdered low car/keto sweetener of your
choice.
1 tsp of vanilla extract, I prefer real vanilla extract.
Imitation vanilla has sugar in the ingredients.

## Directions

Melt the butter in a small saucepan over medium heat.  Add in heavy whipping cream and stir.  Then add in the powdered sweetener and vanilla extract.  Whisk until smooth.  After the donuts have cooled down, spoon or dip the glaze over the donuts.  Let stand a few minutes so the glaze will set.  Then serve.

## Peanut Butter

If it is difficult for you to find a peanut butter with no sugar in the ingredients, here is an easy homemade recipe that does not.

- One jar of roasted peanuts.  Be sure to read the ingredients and nutritional info on the back.
- Put the entire jar of peanuts into a blender or food processor.
- Add salt to taste if you get the unsalted peanuts.
- Pulse for 5 to 10 minutes while occasionally scraping nuts from the sides of the blender.
- You have made peanut butter.

## Saltine Crackers Low Carb Keto

Ingredients

2 cups almond flour
1 egg
1 tbls of butter, melted

½ tsp baking powder
½ tsp salt
1tbls low car sweetener. I use Swerve.
½ tsp butter extract (optional)

## Directions

Pre heat oven to 350 degrees F. In a medium to large mixing bowl mix dry ingredients until well combines. Then add the wet ingredients. Mix until stiff dough forms. Then put dough on parchment paper. Cover the dough with a second piece of parchment paper. Roll out thin. The thinner the crispier they will be. After you have rolled dough to your desired thickness. Trim off edges so the dough will be in a rectangle/square shape. After you have done that, with a pizza cutter cut the dough into small square like a saltine cracker. With a knife of fork, punch 4 to 6 holes in each cracker square. Place in oven for 7 to 8 minutes. Take them out and flip them over. Re arrange then place back into the oven for about five more minutes. Allow them to cool completely when you take them out of the oven.

**Notes:**

# Section 3

# Summary
# &

# Conclusion

## Summary and Conclusion

The information that I have written in this booklet will definitely help get blood sugar and hbA1c to normal. It did for me. Just follow and don't get discouraged. Lowering your numbers can take a little while, sometimes weeks or months. Remember that sometimes no matter what you do, blood sugar seems to have a "mind of its own".

When this happens, stay the course and stick to it. It will come down and you WILL have victory.


## Summary

- Drastically cut carbs and starches out of your diet
- Read ingredients on food packages
- Learn the different names of sugar/starches. When in doubt, look the word up on your phone.
- Most people carry their phone with them.
- Do time restricted eating/intermittent fasting.
- Exercise, a brisk walk for 15 to 30 minutes after meal(s) will help
- No snacking, ok to have an extremely low carb desert occasionally
- Make your last meal of the day no later than 5:30 pm and definitely nothing after 8:00 pm
- Also, the last meal of the day should have fewer carbs/starches than your lunch
- Test just before your meals. Then 1 hour after and then another hour after that.  This will let you know which foods are spiking your blood sugar and which ones won't.  Eliminate the foods that spike your blood sugar.  In other words, eat to your blood sugar meter.
- Get enough sleep.  At least 8 hours.
- Avoid stress as much as possible.

www.ingramcontent.com/pod-product-compliance
Lightning Source LLC
Chambersburg PA
CBHW051710250726
48653CB00007B/2947